MEDITERR

DIET RECIPES

The Healthy Diet Cookbook

for Brain Health and

Prevent Disease

Med Kitchen Academy

No part of this book may be reproduced or transmitted in any form or by any means, electronic or mechanical, including photocopying, recording or by any information storage and retrieval system, without written permission from the author, except for the inclusion of brief quotations in a review.

Limit of Liability and Disclaimer of Warranty: The publisher has used its best efforts in preparing this book, and the information provided herein is provided "as is." This book is designed to provide information and motivation to our readers. It is sold with the understanding that the publisher is not engaged to render any type of psychological, legal, or any other kind of professional advice. The content of each article is the sole expression and opinion of its author, and not necessarily that of the publisher. No warranties or guarantees are expressed or implied by the publisher's choice to include any of the content in this volume. Neither the publisher nor the individual author(s) shall be liable for any physical, psychological, emotional, financial, or commercial damages, including, but not limited to, special, incidental, consequential or other damages. Our views and rights are the same: You are responsible for your own choices, actions, and results.

TABLE OF CONTENTS

The Mediterranean Food Pyramid

The Mediterranean lifestyle follows a very specific food pyramid that is probably a little different than the one you're used to. Certain food groups are given priority while others should be consumed in moderation. Studies have shown that these foods are protective against the effects of certain chronic diseases.

Mediterranean Diet Pyramid

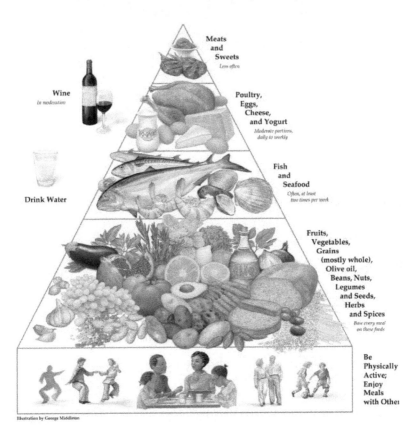

Meats and Sweets
Less often

Wine
In moderation

Poultry, Eggs, Cheese, and Yogurt
Moderate portions, daily to weekly

Fish and Seafood
Often, at least two times per week

Drink Water

Fruits, Vegetables, Grains (mostly whole), Olive oil, Beans, Nuts, Legumes and Seeds, Herbs and Spices
Base every meal on these foods

Be Physically Active; Enjoy Meals with Other

Illustration by George Middleton

Tomato Basil White Bean Salad

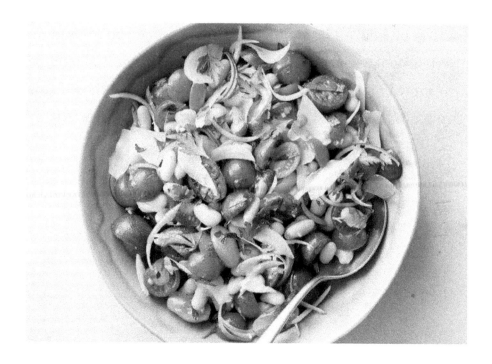

Preparation Time: 10 minutes

Cooking Time: 5 minutes

Serve: 4

Ingredients:

- 1 cup can white beans, drained and rinsed
- 2 tbsp fresh parsley, chopped
- 2 tbsp fresh basil, chopped
- 8.5 oz cherry tomatoes, halved
- 2 lemon juice

- 2 garlic cloves, minced
- 1 small onion, diced
- 3 tbsp olive oil
- Pepper
- Salt

Directions:

In a small bowl, whisk together lemon juice, olive oil, garlic, pepper, and salt. Set aside.

Add remaining ingredients into the mixing bowl and mix well.

Pour dressing over salad and toss well.

Serve and enjoy.

Nutritional Value (Amount per Serving):

Calories 182; Fat 11.4 g; Carbohydrates 16.1 g; Protein 5.1 g; Sugar 3.4 g; Cholesterol 0 mg

Vegan Leek Rice

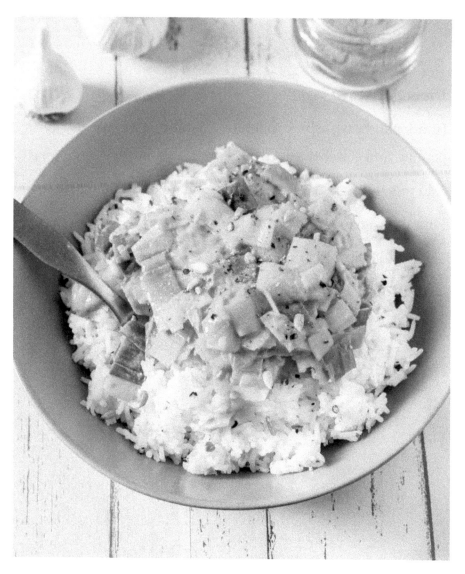

Preparation Time: 10 minutes

Cooking Time: 30 minutes

Serve: 4

Ingredients:

- ½ cup brown rice, uncooked
- 1 ¼ cup hot water
- 1 ½ tsp tomato paste
- 1 ½ tbsp dill, chopped
- 1/3 cup olive oil
- 1 lb leeks, sliced
- Pepper
- Salt

Directions:

Add sliced leek in boiling water and cook for 2-3 minutes. Strain and set aside.

Heat oil in a saucepan over medium-low heat.

Add leek and sauté until softened, about 5-7 minutes.

Add tomato paste and dill and cook for 1-2 minutes.

Add hot water, rice, pepper, and salt and stir well.

Cover the saucepan with a lid and simmer over low heat for 20 minutes.

Serve and enjoy.

Nutritional Value (Amount per Serving):

Calories 304; Fat 17.8 g; Carbohydrates 35.2 g; Protein 3.8 g; Sugar 4.7 g; Cholesterol 0 mg

Flavorful Spinach Rice

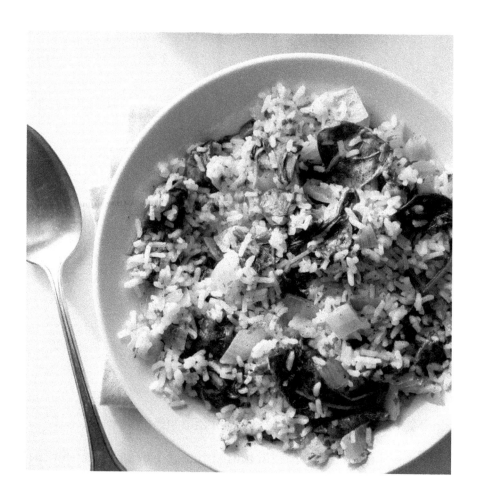

Preparation Time: 10 minutes

Cooking Time: 35 minutes

Serve: 6

Ingredients:

- 1 cup brown rice, uncooked

- ½ tbsp lemon zest
- 1 ½ tbsp fresh lemon juice
- 2 cups vegetable stock
- ½ lb baby spinach
- 3 tbsp dill, chopped
- 4 tbsp green onion, chopped
- 1 tbsp garlic, chopped
- 1 onion, chopped
- 3 tbsp olive oil

Directions:

Heat oil in a large pot over medium-high heat.

Add onion and sauté for 5 minutes or until onion softens.

Add garlic, 2 tbsp green onion, and 2 tbsp dill and sauté for 2 minutes.

Add spinach and cook until spinach is wilted about 3-4 minutes.

Add rice and stock and stir well. Bring to boil.

Turn heat to medium-low and simmer for 20 minutes.

Stir in lemon zest, lemon juice, and remaining green onion and dill.

Serve and enjoy.

Nutritional Value (Amount per Serving):

Calories 201; Fat 8.5 g; Carbohydrates 29.3 g; Protein 4.2 g; Sugar 1.5 g; Cholesterol 0 mg

Quinoa with Chickpeas & Spinach

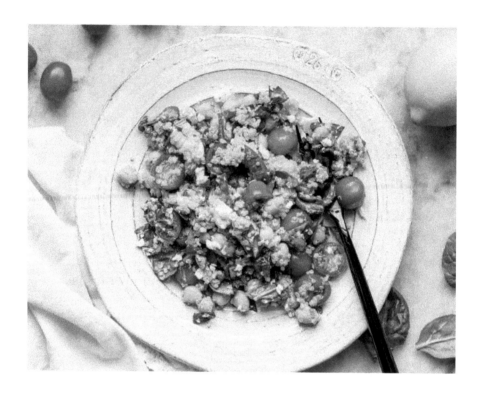

Preparation Time: 10 minutes

Cooking Time: 25 minutes

Serve: 6

Ingredients:

- 1 cup quinoa, uncooked
- 14.5 oz can chickpeas, drained and rinsed
- 1 cup spinach, chopped
- 2 cups vegetable stock

- ½ cup sun-dried tomatoes, chopped
- ¾ cup olives, sliced
- ¼ tsp dried dill
- ¼ tsp dried thyme
- ½ tsp chili flakes
- 2 tbsp shallot, minced
- 1 tbsp garlic, minced
- 1 tbsp olive oil
- Pepper
- **Salt**

Directions:

Heat olive oil in a saucepan over medium heat.

Add shallot, garlic, and chili flakes and cook for 2 minutes.

Add dill and thyme and cook for 30 seconds.

Add quinoa, sun-dried tomatoes, and olives and stir for 30 seconds.

Add stock and stir well. Bring to boil.

Cover and turn heat to low and simmer for 20-25 minutes or until liquid is absorbed.

Remove lid. Add chickpeas and spinach and stir until spinach is wilted.

Season with pepper and salt.

Serve and enjoy.

Nutritional Value (Amount per Serving):

Calories 235; Fat 7 g; Carbohydrates 36.9 g; Protein 8 g; Sugar 0.8 g; Cholesterol 0 mg

Balsamic Balela Mediterranean Medley

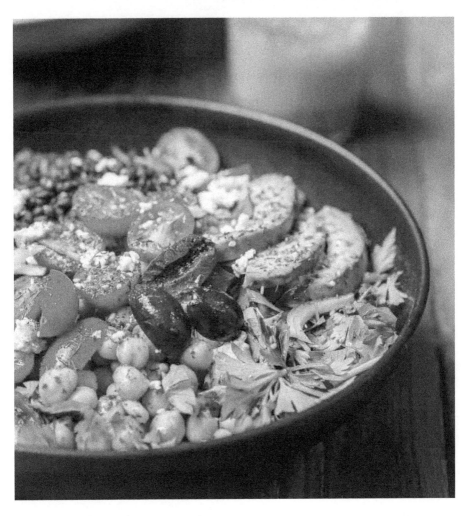

Preparation Time: 15 minutes

Cooking Time: 0 minutes

Servings: 6

Serving Size: 1-cup

Ingredients:

For the Salad:

- 4-pcs green onions, chopped
- 3½-cups chickpeas, cooked
- 2½-cups grape or cherry tomatoes, sliced in halves
- 1-pc jalapeno, finely chopped (optional)
- ½-green bell pepper, cored and chopped
- ½-cup sun-dried tomatoes (preserved in jars with olive oil)
- ½-cup parsley leaves, freshly chopped
- ½-cup mint or basil leaves, freshly chopped
- ⅓-cup Kalamata olives, pitted
- ¼-cup green olives, pitted

For the Dressing:

- Salt and black pepper
- 2-tbsp white wine vinegar
- 2-tbsp lemon juice
- 1-tsp ground sumac
- 1-clove garlic, minced
- ½-tsp red pepper, crushed (optional)
- ½-tsp Aleppo pepper
- ¼-cup extra-virgin olive oil

Directions:

For the Salad:

Combine all the salad ingredients in a large mixing bowl. Mix well until fully combined.

For the Dressing:

Combine and whisk together all the dressing ingredients in a separate smaller mixing bowl. Mix well until fully combined.

Drizzle the dressing over the salad. Toss gently to coat evenly. Cover and refrigerate the salad for 30 minutes before serving.

To serve, give the salad a quick toss. Taste to adjust seasoning, if necessary.

Nutrition: Calories: 228, Total Fats: 3.3g, Dietary Fiber: 10.6g, Carbohydrates: 39.2g, Protein: 12.5g

Lebanese Lemony Fattoush Fusion

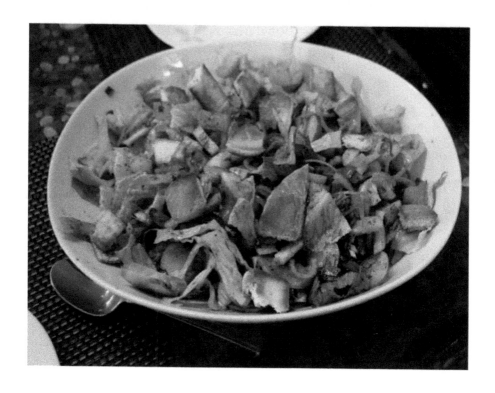

Preparation Time: 10 minutes

Cooking Time: 5 minutes

Servings: 8

Serving Size: 1-serving bowl

Ingredients:

For the Salad:

- 2-loaves whole-wheat pita bread
- 3-tbsp extra-virgin olive oil

- Salt and pepper
- ½-tsp sumac
- 5-pcs Roma tomatoes, chopped
- 5-pcs radishes, stems removed, thinly sliced
- 5-pcs green onions, chopped
- 2-cups fresh parsley leaves, stems removed, chopped
- 1-pc English cucumber, chopped
- 1-heart Romaine lettuce, chopped
- 1-cup fresh mint leaves, chopped (optional)

For the Lime-Vinaigrette Dressing:

- Salt and pepper
- 1-tsp ground sumac or lemon zest
- 1½-lime, juice
- ⅓-cup extra-virgin olive oil
- ¼-tsp ground cinnamon
- ¼-tsp ground allspice

Directions:

For the Salad:

In your toaster oven, toast the pita bread for 2 minutes until turning crisp, but not browned.

Heat 3 tbsp of olive oil in a large frying pan. Cut the toasted pita bread into pieces, and add them in the pan. Fry the broken pita pieces for 3 minutes until browned, tossing frequently.

Season the pita chips with salt, pepper, and sumac. Remove the seasoned pita chips from the heat and place them on paper towels to drain.

Combine the remainder of the salad ingredients in a large mixing bowl. Mix until fully combined.

For the Lime-Vinaigrette Dressing:

Combine and whisk together all the dressing ingredients in a separate smaller mixing bowl. Mix well until fully combined.

Drizzle the lime-vinaigrette dressing over the salad. Toss gently to coat evenly.

Add the oil-drained pita chips and toss gently again until fully combined.

Nutrition: Calories: 478.8, Total Fats: 18.1g, Dietary Fiber: 3.7g, Carbohydrates: 32.1g, Protein: 21.3g

Tasty Tuna Super Salad

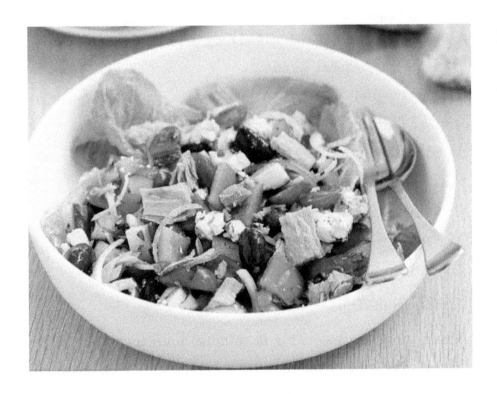

Preparation Time: 15 minutes

Cooking Time: 10 minutes

Servings: 4

Serving Size: 1-cup

Ingredients:

For the Salad:

- 8-oz. fresh green beans, trimmed

- ½-head Romaine lettuce, cored and cut crosswise into ribbons
- 3-tbsp olive oil
- 2-5 oz. cans olive oil-packed tuna, drained
- ½-cup radishes, sliced
- ½-cup black or green olives, pitted
- 1-pc red or yellow sweet pepper, cut into strips

For the Dressing:

- 2-pcs lemons, (1-tbsp. zest, 6-tbsp. juice)
- 4-tsp capers, rinsed
- 2-tsp Dijon-style mustard

Directions:

For the Salad:

Steam the green beans for 10 minutes until they are tender. Remove the beans from the steamer and put them in a bowl of ice water to cool. Strain and drain thoroughly. Set aside.

For the Dressing:

Combine and whisk together all the dressing ingredients in a mixing bowl. Mix well until fully combined.

Arrange the lettuce on a large platter. Top the lettuce bed with the steamed beans, tuna, radishes, olives, and sweet pepper.

Drizzle the dressing over the salad. Toss gently excluding the bed of lettuce to coat evenly.

Nutrition: Calories: 265, Total Fats: 18g, Dietary Fiber: 4g, Carbohydrates: 10g, Protein: 17g

Tabbouleh Tidbits Combo Classic

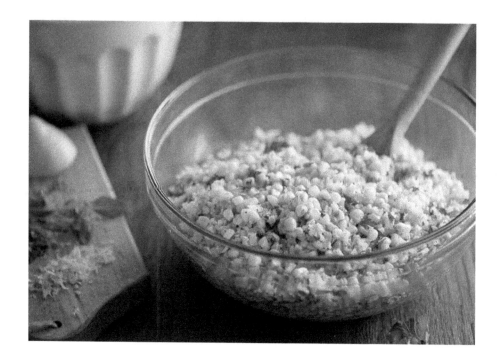

Preparation Time: 20 minutes

Cooking Time: 0 minutes

Servings: 6

Serving Size: 1-cup

Ingredients:

For the Salad:

- ½-cup whole-wheat bulgur
- 4-Roma tomatoes, finely chopped and drained of excess juice
- 4-pcs green onions, very finely chopped

- 2-bunches parsley, stems removed, washed and well-dried, finely chopped
- 1-pc English cucumber, finely chopped
- 12-pcs fresh mint leaves, stems removed, washed, well-dried, finely chopped
- Salt
- Whole-wheat pita bread (optional)
- Romaine lettuce leaves, to serve (optional)

For the Dressing:

- 3-tbsp lemon juice
- 3-tbsp extra-virgin olive oil

Directions:

For the Salad:

Rinse the bulgur and soak in water for 7 minutes. Drain thoroughly by squeezing the bulgur to rid excess water. Set aside.

Combine the remainder of the salad ingredients in a large mixing bowl. Mix until fully combined. Add the bulgur and season with salt. Mix again.

For the Dressing:

Combine and whisk together all the dressing ingredients in a mixing bowl. Mix well until fully combined.

Drizzle the dressing over the salad. Toss gently to coat evenly.

Cover and refrigerate the salad for 30 minutes before serving. If desired, serve the tabbouleh salad with a side dish of whole-wheat pita bread and Romaine lettuce leaves, which serve as 'boats' or wraps for the salad.

Nutrition: Calories: 190, Total Fats: 10g, Dietary Fiber: 3.1g, Carbohydrates: 25.5g, Protein: 3.2g

Athenian Avgolemono Sour Soup

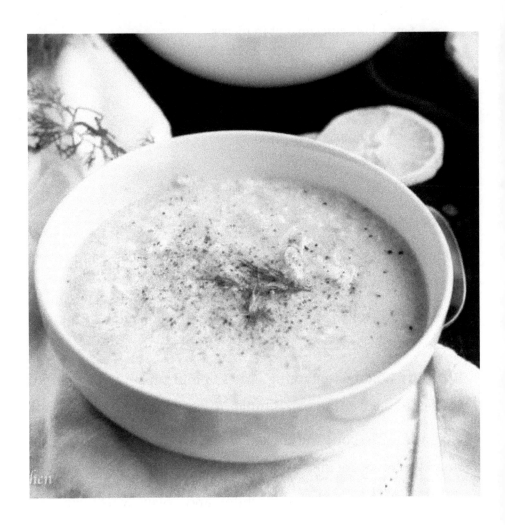

Preparation Time: 20 minutes

Cooking Time: 90 minutes

Servings: 6

Serving Size: 1-cup

Ingredients:

- 8-cups water
- 1-pc whole chicken, cut in pieces
- Salt and pepper
- 1-cup whole grain rice
- 4-pcs eggs, separated
- 2-pcs lemons, juice
- ¼-cup fresh dill, minced
- Dill sprigs and lemon slices for garnish

Directions:

Pour the water in a large pot. Add the chicken pieces, and cover the pot. Simmer for an hour.

Remove the cooked chicken pieces from the pot and take 2-cups of the chicken broth. Set aside and let it cool.

Bring to a boil the remaining. Add salt and pepper to taste. Add the rice and cover the pot. Simmer for 20 minutes.

Meanwhile, de-bone the cooked chicken and tear the flesh into small pieces. Set aside.

Work on the separated egg whites and yolks: whisk the egg whites until stiff; whisk the yolks with the lemon juice.

Pour the egg yolk mixture to the egg white mixture. Whisk well until fully combined. Add gradually the reserved 2-cups of chicken broth to the mixture, whisking constantly to prevent the eggs from curdling.

After fully incorporating the egg mixture and chicken broth, pour this mixture into the simmering broth and rice. Add the dill, and stir well. Simmer further without bringing it to a boil.

Add the chicken pieces to the soup. Mix until fully combined.

To serve, ladle the soup in bowls and sprinkle with fresh ground pepper. Garnish with lemon slices and dill sprigs.

Nutrition: Calories: 122.4, Total Fats: 1.2g, Dietary Fiber: 0.2g, Carbohydrates: 7.5g, Protein: 13.7g

Spring Soup with Gourmet Grains

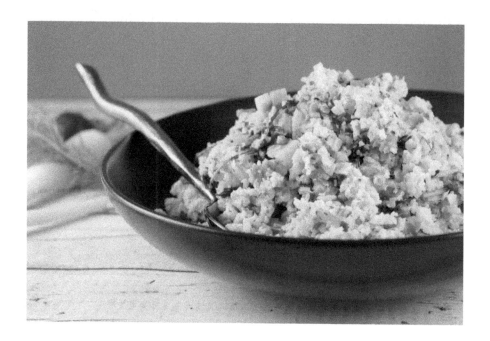

Preparation Time: 10 minutes

Cooking Time: 25 minutes

Servings: 6

Serving Size: 1-cup

Ingredients:

- 2-tbsp olive oil
- 1-pc small onion, diced
- 6-cups chicken broth, homemade (refer to the recipe of Avgolemono Soup)
- 1-bay leaf

- ½-cup of fresh dill, chopped (divided)
- ⅓-cup Italian or Arborio whole grain rice
- 1-cup asparagus, chopped
- 1-cup carrots, diced
- 1½-cups cooked chicken, de-boned and diced or shredded
- ½-lemon, juice
- 1-pc large egg
- 2-tbsp water
- Kosher salt and fresh pepper to taste
- Fresh chives, minced for garnish

Directions:

Heat the olive oil and sauté the onions for 5 minutes in a large stockpot placed over medium heat. Pour in the chicken broth. Add the bay leaf and half of the dill. Bring to a boil.

Add rice and turn the heat to medium-low. Simmer for 10 minutes.

Add the asparagus and carrots. Cook for 15 minutes until the vegetables are tender and the rice cooks through.

Add the cooked shredded chicken. Continue simmer over low heat.

In the meantime, combine the lemon juice and egg with water in a mixing bowl.

Take ½-cup of the simmering stock and pour it on the lemon-egg mixture, whisking gradually to prevent eggs from curdling.

Pour the lemon-egg broth into the stockpot, still whisking gradually. Soon as the soup thickens, turn off heat.

Remove the bay leaf, and discard. Add the remaining dill, salt, and pepper.

To serve, ladle the creamy soup into bowls and garnish with minced chives.

Nutrition: Calories: 252.8, Total Fats: 8g, Dietary Fiber: 0.3g, Carbohydrates: 19.8g, Protein; 25.6g

Spiced Soup with Lentils & Legumes

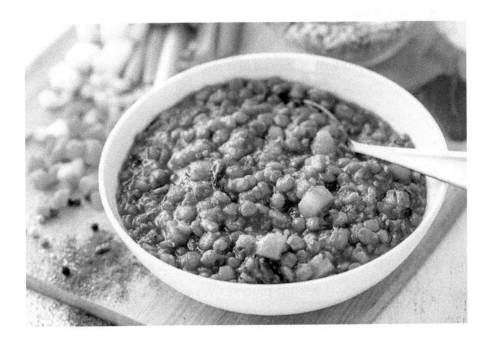

Preparation Time: 15 minutes

Cooking Time: 35 minutes

Servings: 6

Serving Size: 1-cup

Ingredients:

- 2-tbsp extra-virgin olive oil
- 2-cloves garlic, minced
- 4-pcs large celery stalks, diced
- 2-pcs large onions, diced

- 6-cups water
- 1-tsp cumin
- ¾-tsp turmeric
- ½-tsp cinnamon
- ½-tsp fresh ginger, grated
- 1-cup dried lentils, rinsed and sorted
- 1-16-oz. can chickpeas (garbanzo beans), drained and rinsed
- 3-pcs ripe tomatoes, cubed
- ½-lemon, juice
- ½ cup fresh cilantro or parsley, chopped
- Salt

Directions:

Heat the olive oil and sauté the garlic, celery, and onion for 5 minutes in a large stockpot placed over medium heat.

Pour in the water. Add the spices and lentils. Cover the stockpot and simmer for 40 minutes until the lentils are tender.

Add the chickpeas and tomatoes. (Pour more water and additional spices, if desired.) Simmer for 15 minutes over low heat.

Pour in the lemon juice and stir the soup. Add the cilantro or parsley and salt to taste.

Nutrition: Calories: 123, Total Fats: 3g, Dietary Fiber: 5g, Carbohydrates: 19g, Protein: 5g

Mediterranean Spaghetti

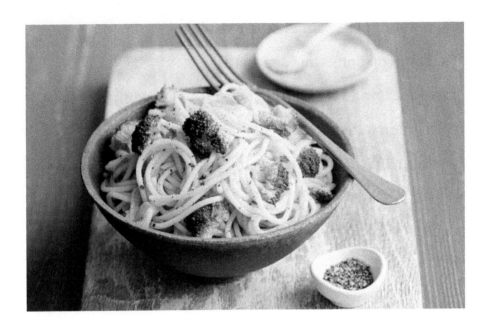

Preparation time: 10 minutes

Cooking time: 10 minutes

Servings: 2

Ingredients:

- 1/3 cup broccoli

- 7 oz whole grain spaghetti

- 2 oz Parmesan, shaved

- ½ teaspoon ground black pepper

- 1 cup water, for cooking

Directions:

Chop the broccoli into the small florets.

Pour water in the pan. Bring it to boil.

Add broccoli florets and spaghetti.

Close the lid and cook the ingredients for 10 minutes.

Then drain water.

Add ground black pepper and shaved Parmesan. Shake the spaghetti well.

Nutrition: calories 430, fat 8.8, fiber 9.3, carbs 72.4, protein 23.6

Hummus Pasta

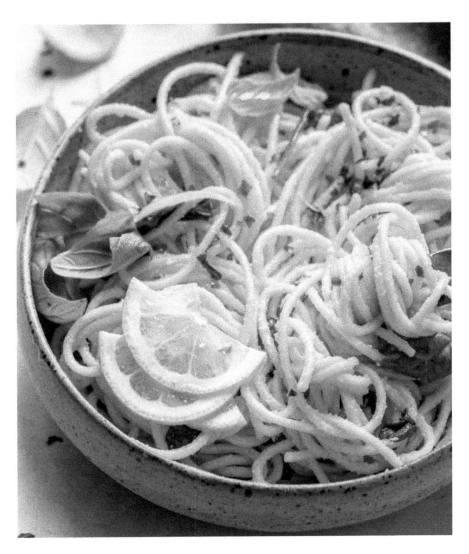

Preparation time: 10 minutes

Cooking time: 15 minutes

Servings: 4

Ingredients:

- 10 oz soba noodles
- ½ teaspoon Italian seasoning
- ¼ teaspoon sage
- ¾ teaspoon ground coriander
- 4 teaspoons hummus
- 1 teaspoon butter, softened
- 2 cups water, for cooking

Directions:

Pour water in the pan. Bring the liquid to boil.

Add soba noodles, sage, and ground coriander.

Boil the noodles for 15 minutes over the medium-high heat. The cooked soba noodles should be tender.

Then drain water.

Mix up together soba noodles, butter, and Italian seasoning.

Place the cooked pasta in the bowls and top with hummus.

Nutrition: calories 256, fat 2.1, fiber 0.3, carbs 53.6, protein 10.6

Mushroom and Garlic Spaghetti

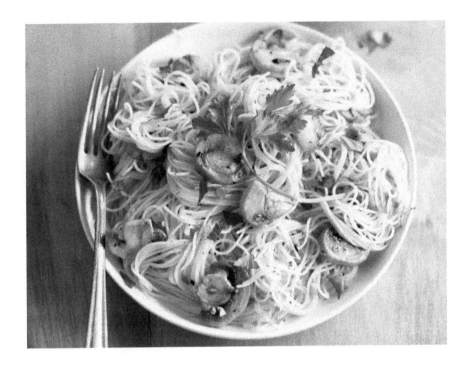

Preparation time: 10 minutes

Cooking time: 20 minutes

Servings: 4

Ingredients:

- ½ cup white mushrooms, chopped

- 3 garlic cloves, diced

- 2 tablespoons sesame oil

- ½ teaspoon chili flakes

- 1 teaspoon salt

- 1 teaspoon dried marjoram

- 10 oz whole grain buckwheat spaghetti

- 1 cup water, for cooking

Directions:

Pour sesame oil in the skillet and heat it up.

Add mushrooms and garlic. Mix up well.

Sprinkle the vegetables with chili flakes, salt, and dried marjoram.

Pour water in the pan and bring to boil.

Add buckwheat spaghetti and cook them according to the direction of the manufacturer.

Drain water from spaghetti and transfer them in the mushroom mixture.

Mix up spaghetti well and cook for 5 minutes over the medium-low heat.

Nutrition: calories 303, fat 8.7, fiber 5.2, carbs 52.4, protein 10.4

Pasta with Creamy Sauce

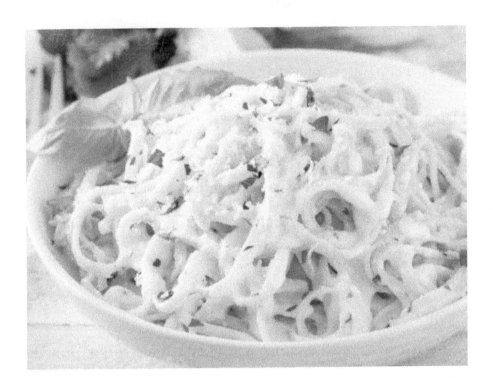

Preparation time: 10 minutes

Cooking time: 7 minutes

Servings: 2

Ingredients:

- 7 oz quinoa pasta

- 1 tablespoon fresh dill, chopped

- 1 tablespoon fresh cilantro, chopped

- ½ teaspoon ground black pepper
- 1 oz Parmesan, grated
- ½ cup milk
- 1 cup water, for cooking

Directions:

Pour water in the pan and bring it to boil.

Add quinoa pasta and boil it for 2 minutes. Drain the water.

Sprinkle pasta with dill, cilantro, and ground black pepper.

Then bring to boil milk and mix it up with Parmesan. Stir well until cheese is melted.

Pour the milk sauce over the pasta.

Nutrition: calories 252, fat 6.3, fiber 2.8, carbs 39, protein 10.9

Feta Macaroni

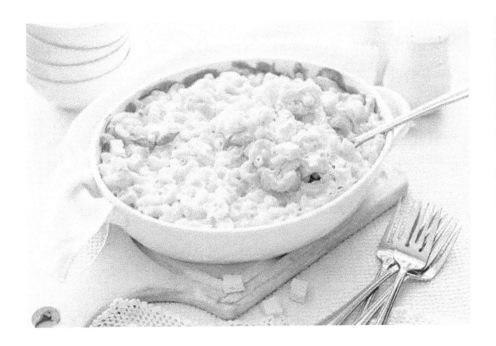

Preparation time: 15 minutes

Cooking time: 25 minutes

Servings: 4

Ingredients:

- 5 oz whole grain macaroni

- 4 oz Feta cheese, crumbled

- 2 eggs, beaten

- ½ teaspoon chili pepper

- 1 teaspoon almond butter

- 1 cup water, for cooking

Directions:

Mix up together water and macaroni and boil according to the directions of the manufacturer.

Then drain water.

Add almond butter, chili pepper, and Feta cheese. Mix up well.

Transfer the mixture in the casserole mold and flatten well.

Pour beaten eggs over the macaroni and bake for 10 minutes at 355F.

Nutrition: calories 262, fat 11.4, fiber 4.2, carbs 27.2, protein 13.9

Caprese Pasta Salad

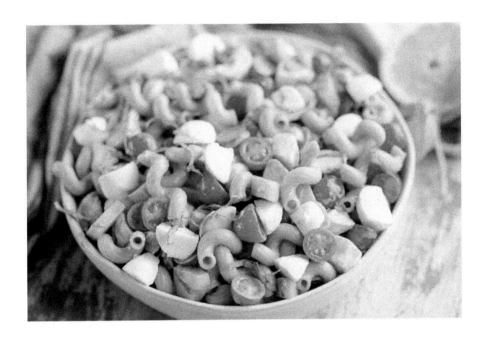

Preparation time: 10 minutes

Cooking time: 15 minutes

Servings: 2

Ingredients:

- 2 oz whole grain elbow macaroni

- 1 tablespoon fresh basil

- ¼ cup cherry size Mozzarella

- ½ cup cherry tomatoes, halved

- 1 tablespoon olive oil

- 1 teaspoon dried marjoram

- 1 cup water, for cooking

Directions:

Boil elbow macaroni in water for 15 minutes. Drain water and chill macaroni little.

Chop fresh basil roughly and place it in the salad bowl.

Add Mozzarella, cherry tomatoes, dried marjoram, olive oil, and macaroni.

Mix up salad well.

Nutrition: calories 170, fat 9.7, fiber 1.1, carbs 15, protein 6

Basil Buckwheat Pasta

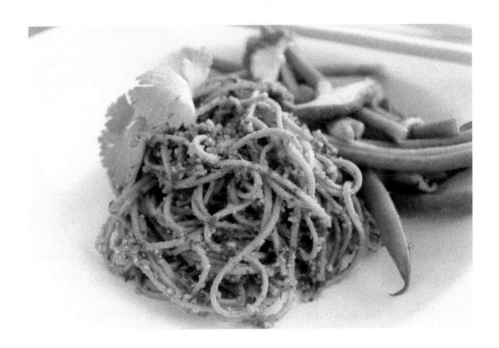

Preparation time: 8 minutes

Cooking time: 20 minutes

Servings: 4

Ingredients:

- 1 cup fresh basil
- 8 oz buckwheat pasta
- ½ teaspoon salt
- 1 tablespoon almonds, chopped
- ½ oz Parmesan, grated

- ½ teaspoon dried oregano

- ¾ teaspoon chili pepper

- ½ teaspoon coconut oil

- 1 cup water, for cooking

Directions:

Bring the water to boil and add pasta.

Boil it for 10 minutes. Drain water.

After this, toss coconut oil in the skillet and melt it.

Put in the blender: salt, almonds, Parmesan, oregano, chili pepper, and fresh basil. Blend until the mixture is smooth.

Add the basil mixture in the hot coconut oil and roast for 2 minutes.

Then add cooked buckwheat pasta and mix up well.

Cook the meal for 3 minutes more.

Nutrition: calories 247, fat 3.3, fiber 3.4, carbs 50.8, protein 9.7

Tomato Pasta Fagioli

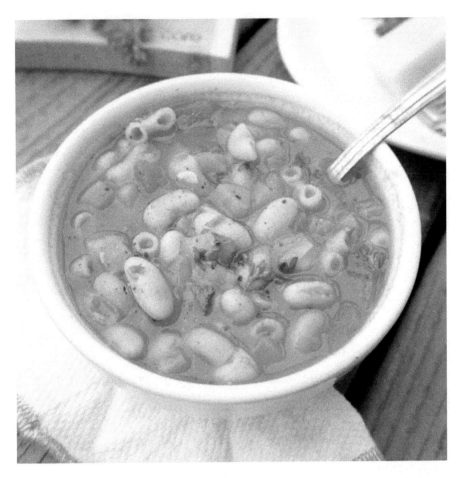

Preparation time: 7 minutes

Cooking time: 10 minutes

Servings: 4

Ingredients:

- 3 oz red kidney beans, canned

- 1 teaspoon tomato paste

- 7 oz quinoa pasta

- 1 tomato, chopped

- 1 teaspoon olive oil

- ¼ yellow onion, diced

- 1/3 carrot, chopped

- 1 teaspoon almond butter

- 1 cup water, for cooking

Directions:

Place almond butter in the skillet and melt it.

Add chopped carrot, tomato, and yellow onion. Cook the vegetables for 7 minutes over the medium heat. Stir them from time to time.

Meanwhile, bring the water to boil. Add quinoa pasta and cook it for 2 minutes over the medium heat. Drain the water.

Add pasta in the vegetable mixture.

Then add tomato paste, red kidney beans, and olive oil.

Cook the pasta for 5 minutes over the high heat. Stir it with the help of the spatula every 1 minute.

Nutrition: calories 267, fat 5.5, fiber 6.3, carbs 46.4, protein 9.5

Chewy Barley

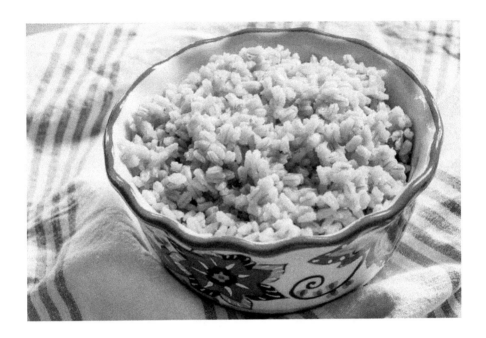

Preparation time: 6 minutes

Cooking time: 25 minutes

Servings: 2

Ingredients:

- 1/3 cup barley

- 4 oz beef broth

- ½ teaspoon salt

- ¾ teaspoon curry paste

- 1 teaspoon sesame oil

Directions:

Place barley and beef broth in the pan.

Add salt, curry paste, and sesame oil.

Mix up the ingredients until curry paste is dissolved.

Then close the lid and bring it to boil.

Boil the barley with the closed lid for 20 minutes.

Nutrition: calories 150, fat 4.4, fiber 5.3, carbs 23.3, protein 5.1

Wild Rice Stew

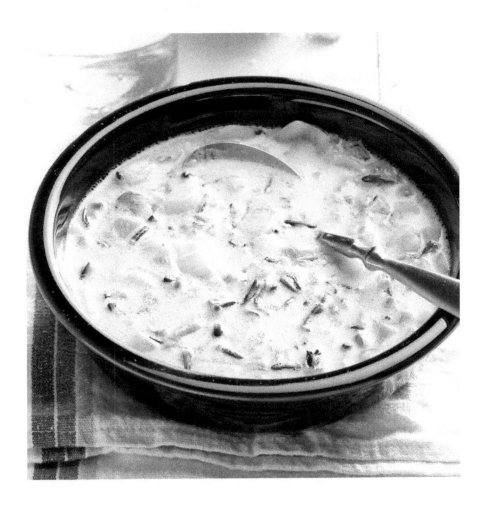

Preparation time: 10 minutes

Cooking time: 40 minutes

Servings: 5

Ingredients:

- 1 cup long grain brown rice (wild rice)
- 3 oz leek, chopped
- 1 white onion, diced
- 1 teaspoon turmeric
- 1 carrot, peeled, chopped
- ½ teaspoon chili flakes
- 3 cups chicken stock
- 1 teaspoon salt
- 1 eggplant, chopped
- 1 tablespoon olive oil
- 2 cups of water

Directions:

Pour olive oil in the skillet.

Add eggplant and roast it for 3 minutes over the medium heat.

Then transfer the vegetables in the pan.

Place onion and leek in the skillet. Roast them for 3 minutes. Stir them from time to time.

Transfer the roasted vegetables in the pan too.

After this, roast carrot for 4 minutes and transfer it in the pan too.

Add brown rice, turmeric, chili flakes, chicken stock, salt, and water in the pan.

Mix up the stew mixture and close the lid.

Simmer the stew for 30 minutes over the medium-low heat.

Nutrition: calories 217, fat 4.4, fiber 5.7, carbs 40.8, protein 4.8

Pumpkin Puree

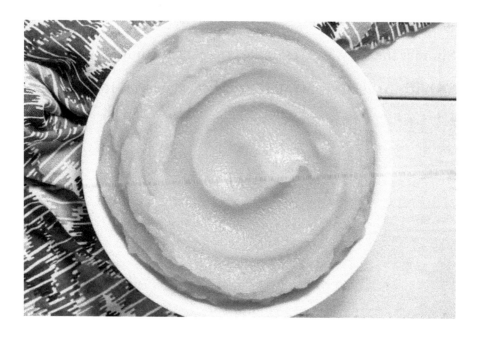

Preparation time: 10 minutes

Cooking time: 30 minutes

Servings: 4

Ingredients:

- 10 oz pumpkin, peeled
- ½ teaspoon butter
- ¾ teaspoon ground ginger
- 1/3 teaspoon salt

Directions:

Chop the pumpkin into the cubes and bake in the preheated to the 360F oven for 30 minutes or until the pumpkin is soft.

After this, transfer the pumpkin cubes in the food processor.

Add butter, salt, and ground ginger.

Blend the vegetable until you get puree or use the potato masher for this step.

Nutrition: calories 30, fat 0.7, fiber 2.1, carbs 6, protein 0.8

Cauliflower Rice

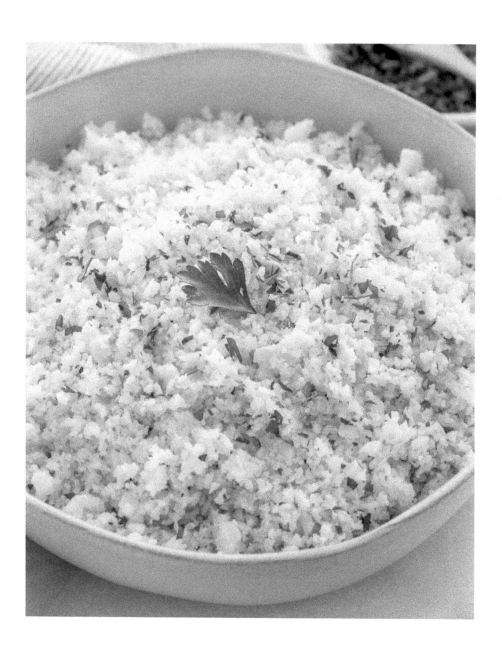

Preparation time: 10 minutes

Cooking time: 10 minutes

Servings: 2

Ingredients:

- 7 oz cauliflower
- 1 teaspoon peanut butter
- ¼ teaspoon chili pepper
- 1 tablespoon fresh dill, chopped
- 1/3 cup beef broth

Directions:

Shred cauliflower until you get cauliflower rice.

Toss peanut butter in the saucepan and melt it.

Add shredded cauliflower. Sprinkle it with chili pepper and dill. Mix up well.

Roast the cauliflower for 2 minutes.

Then add beef broth and bring the mixture to boil.

Simmer the side dish for 3 minutes over the medium heat.

Nutrition: calories 51, fat 1.8, fiber 2.9, carbs 6.9, protein 3.8

Broccoli Puree

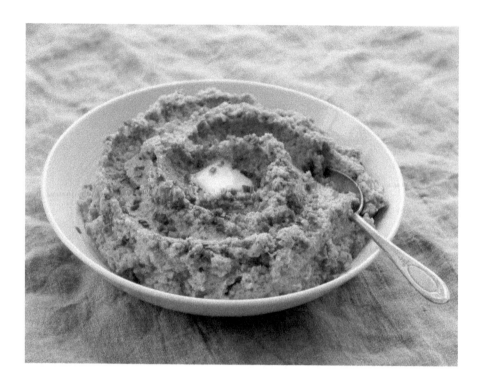

Preparation time: 10 minutes

Cooking time: 15 minutes

Servings: 6

Ingredients:

- 1-pound broccoli, trimmed

- 1 cup chicken stock

- 1 teaspoon butter

- 1 teaspoon salt

Directions:

Line the baking tray with baking paper.

Cut the broccoli into the florets and place them on the baking paper.

Sprinkle them with salt and bake for 10 minutes at 360F.

Meanwhile, pour chicken stock in the pan and bring it to boil.

Add baked cauliflower florets and boil them until soft.

Then drain ½ part of chicken stock. You can leave less liquid if the broccoli is juicy.

Mash the broccoli until you get a soft and fluffy texture.

Add butter and mix up with the help of the spoon.

Nutrition: calories 33, fat 1, fiber 2, carbs 5.1, protein 2.2

Swiss Cheese Pasta

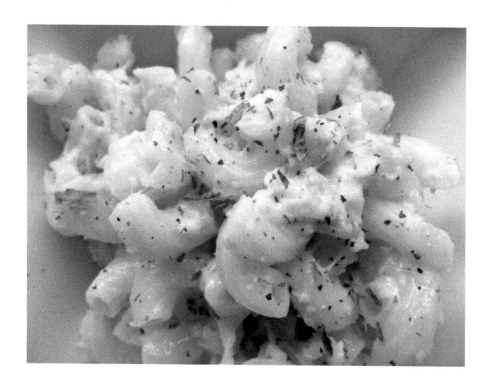

Preparation time: 10 minutes

Cooking time: 15 minutes

Servings: 2

Ingredients:

- 4 oz whole grain pasta

- 1 oz Swiss cheese, shredded

- 1 tablespoon mascarpone

- ½ teaspoon salt

- 1 cup water, for cooking

Directions:

Boil pasta in water for 15 minutes.

Then drain water.

Add salt and mascarpone. Mix up pasta carefully with the help of the spoon.

Add shredded cheese and shake it gently.

The pasta is cooked when the cheese is melted.

Nutrition: calories 186, fat 6.1, fiber 4, carbs 23.1, protein 9.8

Tortellini Salad

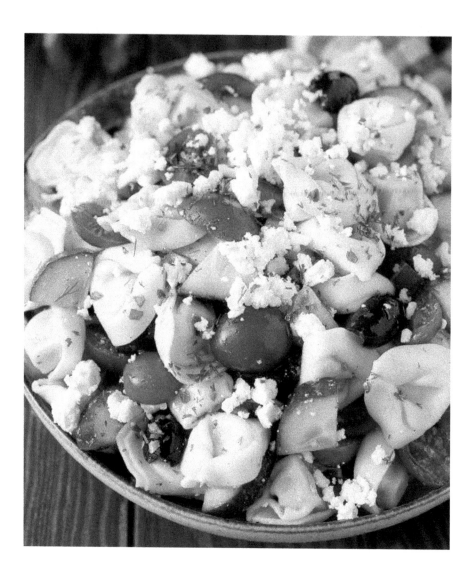

Preparation time: 10 minutes

Cooking time: 15 minutes

Servings: 6

Ingredients:

- 7 oz tortellini
- 3 oz Feta cheese, crumbled
- 5 kalamata olives, chopped
- 1 bell pepper, chopped
- 1/3 cup fresh cilantro, chopped
- 1 tablespoon sesame oil
- ½ teaspoon sesame seeds
- 1 teaspoon fresh basil, chopped
- 1 teaspoon salt
- 1 cup water, for cooking

Directions:

Bring the water to boil, add tortellini, and cook them according to the directions of the manufacturer.

Then drain water and cool tortellini.

Add kalamata olives, chopped bell pepper, cilantro, sesame seeds, sesame oil, basil, and salt.

Then add Feta cheese.

Shake the salad well.

Nutrition: calories 173, fat 8.7, fiber 1.7, carbs 16.8, protein 7.3

Bacon Linguine Pasta

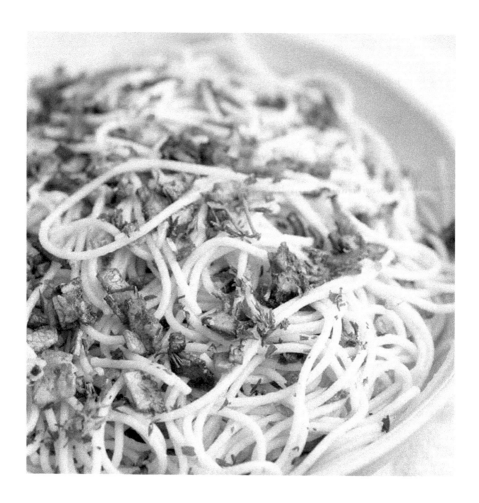

Preparation time: 10 minutes

Cooking time: 20 minutes

Servings: 4

Ingredients:

- 1 egg, beaten

- 4 oz linguine

- 1 oz bacon, chopped

- ½ teaspoon canola oil

- 1 cup cherry tomatoes, halved

- 1 oz Romano cheese, grated

- 1 oz shallot, chopped

- 2 cups of water

Directions:

Pour water in the pan and bring to boil.

Add linguine and cook it according to the directions of the manufacturer.

When the linguine is cooked, drain ½ part of water.

Put bacon in the skillet, add canola oil, and roast it for 5 minutes or until crunchy.

Add cooked bacon in the linguine.

Then add shallot, grated Romano cheese, cherry tomatoes, and beaten egg.

Mix up the pasta carefully until it is homogenous and egg is dissolved.

Simmer pasta for 3 minutes over the medium-low heat.

Nutrition: calories 182, fat 7.3, fiber 0.5, carbs 18.9, protein 10.1

Kingly Kalamata Karithopita

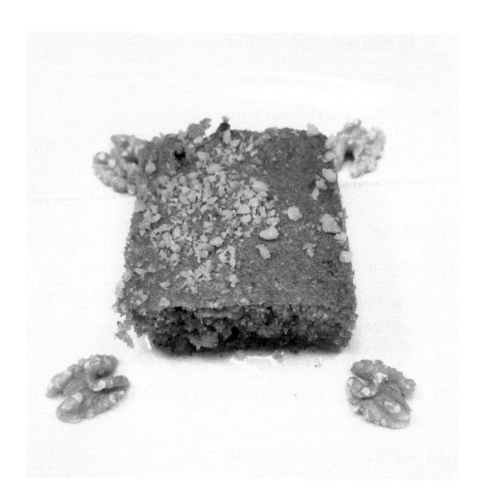

Preparation Time: 15 minutes

Cooking Time: 40 minutes

Servings: 16

Serving Size: 1-slice

Ingredients:

For the Karithopita (Walnut Cake with Syrup):

- 1¼-cups whole-wheat flour
- 1-tsp ground cinnamon
- 1-tsp baking powder
- ¾-cup white sugar
- ½-tsp salt
- ¼-tsp ground cloves
- ⅓-cup extra-virgin olive oil (as shortening)
- ¾-cup milk
- 1-pc egg, whisked
- 1-cup walnuts, finely chopped

For the Honey-Lemon Syrup:

- ¼-cup white sugar
- ¼-cup water
- 1-tsp lemon juice
- ¼-cup honey

Directions:

1. Preheat your oven to 350 °F. Prepare a greased 9" x 9" baking pan. Set aside.

2. Combine and mix the first six Karithopita ingredients in a medium-sized mixing bowl. Mix well until fully incorporated. Transfer the mixture in the mixing bowl of your stand mixer.

3. Pour in the oil, milk, and the egg. Beat the mixture on low speed for 1 minute to a creamy and thick consistency, scraping the bottom of the mixing bowl once to avoid lumps.

4. Stir in the chopped walnuts manually using a spatula. Transfer the batter in the prepared baking pan and spread evenly.

5. Place the pan in the preheated oven. Bake for 40 minutes until an inserted toothpick into the center of the walnut cake comes out clean.

6. Let the walnut cake in the pan cool for 30 minutes. In the meantime, prepare the honey lemon syrup.

For the Lemon Honey-Syrup:

7. Stir in the white sugar with water in a saucepan placed over medium heat. Bring the mixture to a boil. Reduce the heat to low, and allow simmering for 5 minutes.

8. Stir in the lemon juice and honey. Remove the saucepan from the heat.

9. By using a knife, make small slashes in a diamond pattern on the top of the cake. Pour the hot syrup over the walnut cake.

Nutrition: Calories: 198, Total Fats: 9.8g, Dietary Fiber: 0.9g, Carbohydrates: 26.1g, Protein: 2.9g

Apple Applied Cinnamon Cake Cooked with Olive Oil

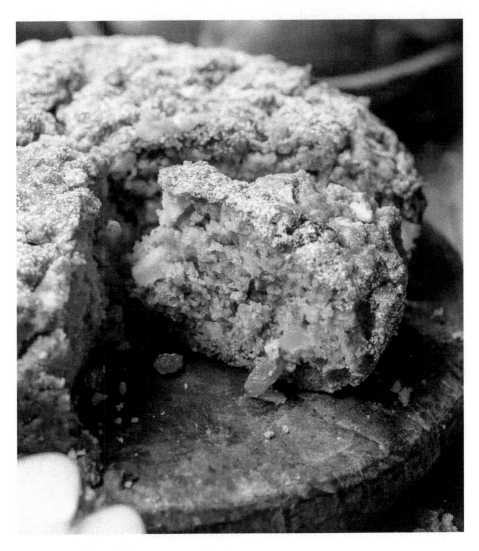

Preparation Time: 20 minutes

Cooking Time: 60 minutes

Servings: 12-slices, Serving Size: 1-slice

Ingredients:

- 4-eggs
- 1-cup brown sugar +2-tbsp for apples
- 1-cup extra-virgin olive oil (as shortening)
- 1-cup milk
- 2-tsp baking powder
- 2½-cups whole-wheat flour
- 1-tsp vanilla extract
- 4-pcs apples, peeled, cored, halved, and sliced thinly
- 1½-tsp ground cinnamon
- ½-cup walnuts, chopped
- ½-cup raisins
- 3-tbsp sesame seeds

Directions:

1. Preheat your oven to 375 °F. Prepare a greased 9" x 9" baking pan. Set aside.

2. By using your electric hand mixer, beat the eggs and a cup of sugar for 10 minutes. Pour in the olive oil and beat the mixture for 3 minutes.

3. Pour in the milk, and add the baking powder, wheat flour, and vanilla. Beat the mixture for another 3 minutes.

4. Transfer half of the batter in the prepared baking pan and spread evenly.

5. Combine and mix the apples, cinnamon, walnuts, raisins, and the 2-tbsp of brown sugar in a mixing bowl. Mix thoroughly until fully combined.

6. Transfer the apple mixture over the batter in the baking pan and spread evenly.

7. Top the apple mixture with the remaining batter. Sprinkle the batter with the sesame seeds.

8. Place the pan in the preheated oven. Bake for 50 minutes until an inserted toothpick into the center of the apple-cinnamon cake comes out clean.

Nutrition: Calories: 420, Total Fats: 23.3g, Dietary Fiber: 3.5g, Carbohydrates: 49.6g, Protein: 7.3g

Naturally Nutty & Buttery Banana Bowl

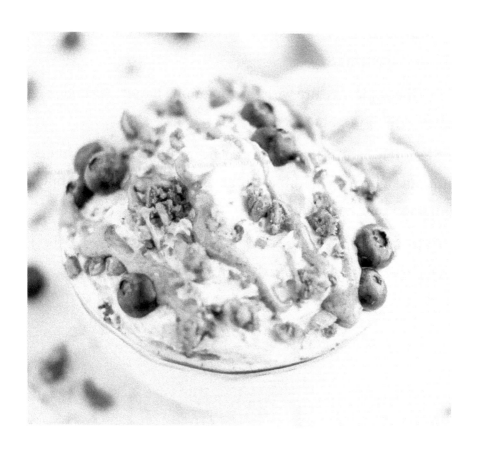

Preparation Time: 5 minutes

Cooking Time: 0 minutes

Servings: 4

Serving Size: 1-cup

Ingredients:

- 4-cups vanilla Greek yogurt
- 2-pcs medium-sized bananas, sliced
- ¼-cup creamy and natural peanut butter
- 1-tsp ground nutmeg
- ¼-cup flaxseed meal

Directions:

1. Divide the yogurt equally between four serving bowls. Top each yogurt bowl with the banana slices.

2. Place the peanut butter in a microwave-safe bowl. Melt the peanut butter in your microwave for 40 seconds. Drizzle one tablespoon of the melted peanut butter over the bananas for each bowl.

3. To serve, sprinkle over with the ground nutmeg and flax-seed meal.

Nutrition: Calories: 370, Total Fats: 10.6g, Dietary Fiber: 4.7g, Carbohydrates: 47.7g, Protein: 22.7g

Queenly Quinoa Choco Crunch Baked Bars

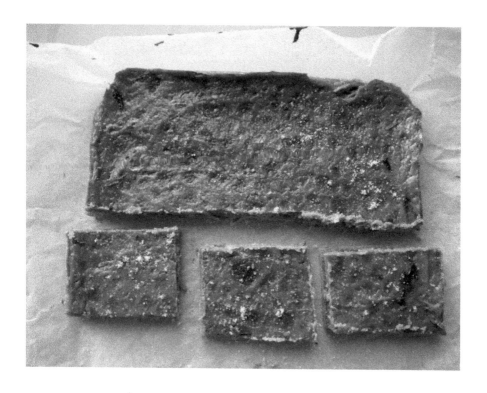

Preparation Time: 5 minutes

Cooking Time: 20 minutes

Servings: 10

Serving Size: 2-square bars

Ingredients:

- 2½-tbsp peanut butter with roasted peanuts
- 2-tbsp water

- 1-lb. semi-sweet chocolate bars, chopped into small pieces
- 1-cup dry quinoa
- ½-tsp vanilla
- 1-tbsp natural peanut butter

Directions:

1. Preheat for 10 minutes a heavy-bottomed pot placed over medium-high heat.

2. Meanwhile, prepare a baking sheet lined with parchment paper. Set aside.

3. Make a peanut butter drizzle by stirring the peanut butter with roasted peanuts with water in a small mixing bowl until fully incorporated. Set aside.

4. Add the quinoa by batch, ¼-cup at a time to pop. Allow each batch to sit at the bottom of the pot, stirring occasionally. Once the quinoa starts to pop, swirl it constantly for 1 minute until the popping subsides. (This can happen too quickly, so ensure to take it off lest the quinoa turns brown.) Set aside.

5. Place the chopped chocolate bars in a microwave-safe mixing bowl. Melt it in your microwave for 30 seconds.

6. Add the popped quinoa, vanilla, and peanut butter in the mixing bowl of the melted chocolate. Mix thoroughly until fully combined.

7. Transfer the chocolate-quinoa mixture in the prepared baking sheet. You need not spread the mixture across the sheet; else, it gets too thin. Simply form a roughly square shape of the mixture, about half an inch thick, in the middle of the sheet.

8. Pour the peanut butter drizzle over chocolate-quinoa square. By using a spatula, spread gently the drizzle entirely around the square.

9. Refrigerate the mixture for an hour until it becomes completely a firm cake. To serve, slice the cake into small square bars.

Nutrition: Calories: 170, Total Fats: 8g, Dietary Fiber: 3g, Carbohydrates: 24g, Protein: 4g

Phyllo Pastry Balkan Baklava

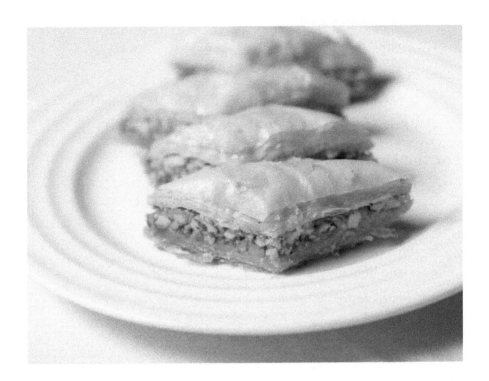

Preparation Time: 30 minutes

Cooking Time: 35 minutes

Servings: 18

Serving Size: 1-slice

Ingredients:

For the Baklava:

- 12-sheets phyllo pastry dough
- 1-tsp ground cloves

- 2-tsp ground cinnamon
- 2-cups walnuts, chopped
- 1-cup sesame seeds
- 2-cups almonds, chopped
- 3-tbsp honey
- 1-cup extra-virgin olive oil (for brushing the dough)
- 18-pcs whole cloves (1 for each piece of baklava slice)

For the Honey Syrup:

- 1 pc lemon, rind
- 1-cinnamon stick
- 2-cups sugar
- 1-cup honey
- 2-cups water
- 1-pc lemon, juice

Directions:

For the Baklava:

1. Preheat your oven to 350 °F.

2. Mix the ground cloves, cinnamon, walnuts, sesame seeds and almonds with honey in a mixing bowl.

3. Brush with olive oil 4-sheets of phyllo pastry, on both sides of each. Lay the oiled sheets on top of each other in a 9" x 9" baking pan.

4. Transfer half of the nut mixture on top of the oiled sheets and spread evenly.

5. Brush with olive oil another set of 4-sheets of phyllo pastry, on both sides. Lay this set of oiled sheets over the nut mixture.

6. Empty the mixing bowl with the remaining nut mixture over the oiled sheets and spread evenly. Top the nut mixture with the last set of 4-sheets of phyllo pastry, brushed in the same manner as the other previous sets.

7. Slice the baklava into 18-equally sized pieces. Top each slice with one whole clove.

8. Place the baking pan in the preheated oven. Bake for 35 minutes until the top turns golden brown. Prepare for the honey syrup while the baklava is baking.

For the Honey Syrup:

9. Combine the lemon peel, cinnamon stick, and sugar with honey and water in a saucepan placed over medium heat. Bring the mixture to a boil. Reduce the heat to low, and simmer for 15 minutes. Let the syrup to cool down before stirring in the lemon juice.

10. Take the baklava out from the oven. To serve, pour over the honey syrup generously over the baklava.

Nutrition: Calories: 482, Total Fats: 24.4g, Dietary Fiber: 4.6g, Carbohydrates: 56.2g, Protein: 6g

Potpourri of Plum, Pistachios & Pomegranate

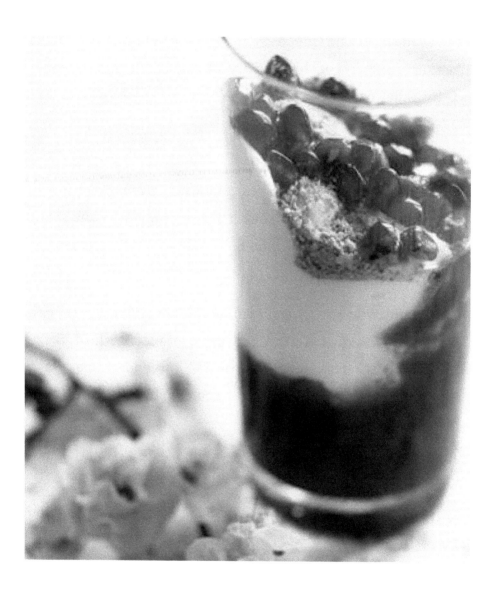

Preparation Time: 30 minutes

Cooking Time: 30 minutes

Servings: 12-servings (3-cups), Serving Size: ¼-cup

Ingredients:

- Olive oil mist
- 1½-cups pistachios, unsalted
- ½-cup dried apricots, chopped
- ¼-cup pomegranate seeds
- ¼-tsp ground nutmeg
- ¼-tsp ground allspice
- ½-tsp cinnamon
- 2-tsp sugar

Directions:

1. Preheat your oven to 350 °F.

2. Spread the pistachios evenly in a rimmed baking sheet misted with olive oil. Bake for 7 minutes until lightly toasted. Let the roasted pistachios to cool completely.

3. Toss the roasted pistachios with the apricots, pomegranate seeds, nutmeg, allspice, cinnamon, and sugar until fully coated.

TIP: You can make this recipe ahead up to 3 days before eating. This dessert recipe is also ideal for solo snacks or as a topping on a cup of yogurt

Nutrition: Calories: 110, Total Fats: 7.1g, Dietary Fiber: 2.1g, Carbohydrates: 11g, Protein: 3.5g

Grecian "Golden Delicious" Dessert

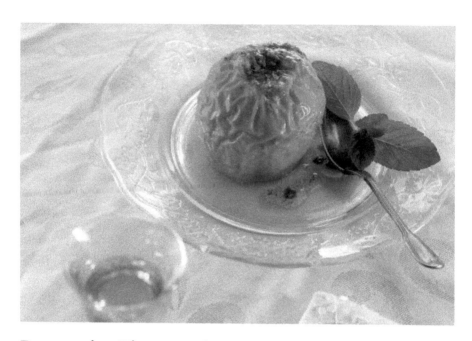

Preparation Time: 10 minutes

Cooking Time: 35 minutes

Servings: 8

Serving Size: 1-slice

Ingredients:

- 1½-lbs. Golden Delicious apples, peeled, cored, and sliced thinly (divided)
- 2-pcs eggs
- Zest of lemon, grated
- ⅓-cup brown sugar
- A pinch of salt

- ¼-cup plus 1-tbsp low-fat milk
- 3-tsp baking powder
- 1 cup less 1-tbsp whole-wheat flour, sifted
- 1-tbsp light brown sugar for topping (optional)
- 1-tbsp icing sugar for dusting

Directions:

1. Preheat your oven to 350 °F. Prepare a greased and flour-sprinkled 8" x 8" baking pan. Set aside.

2. Combine and mix the eggs, lemon zest, sugar, and salt in the mixing bowl of your stand mixer. Beat to a creamy and thick consistency.

3. Pour in the milk, and add the baking powder and flour. Beat until fully incorporated.

4. Add ⅔ or 1-pound of the sliced apples to the batter. By using a spatula, mix thoroughly until fully combined. Transfer the batter in the prepared baking pan.

5. Top the batter with the remaining apple slices. If desired, sprinkle with a tablespoon of brown sugar.

6. Place the pan in the preheated oven. Bake for 35 minutes until an inserted toothpick into the center of the apple cake comes out clean.

7. To serve, dust the low-fat cake with icing sugar.

Nutrition: Calories: 116| Total Fats: 1g, Dietary Fiber: 1.8g, Carbohydrates: 25.3g, Protein: 2.4g

Chocolate Covered Strawberries

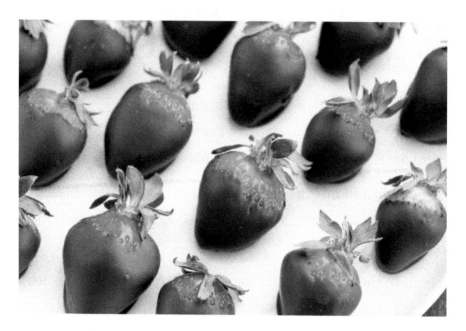

Preparation time: 15 Minutes

Servings: 24 servings

Ingredients:

- 16 ounces milk chocolate chips
- 2 tablespoons shortening
- 1-pound fresh strawberries with leaves

Directions:

In a bain-marie, melt chocolate and shorter, occasionally stirring until smooth. Hold them by the toothpicks and immerse the strawberries in the chocolate mixture.

Put toothpicks in the top of the strawberries.

Turn the strawberries and put the toothpick in the Styrofoam so that the chocolate cools.

Nutrition: 115 calories; 7.3 g of fat; 12.7 g of carbohydrates; 1.4 g of protein; 6 mg cholesterol; 31 mg of sodium

Strawberry Angel Food Dessert

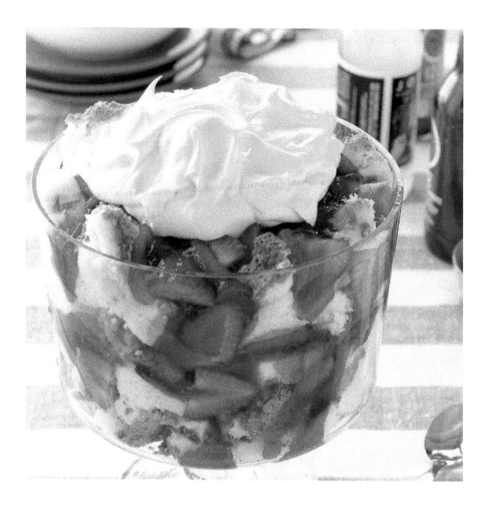

Preparation time: 15 minutes

Servings: 18 servings

Ingredients:

- 1 angel cake (10 inches)

- 2 packages of softened cream cheese
- 1 cup of white sugar, 1 container (8 oz) of frozen fluff, thawed
- 1 liter of fresh strawberries, sliced
- 1 jar of strawberry icing

Directions:

Crumble the cake in a 9 x 13-inch dish.

Beat the cream cheese and sugar in a medium bowl until the mixture is light and fluffy. Stir in the whipped topping. Crush the cake with your hands, and spread the cream cheese mixture over the cake.

Combine the strawberries and the frosting in a bowl until the strawberries are well covered. Spread over the layer of cream cheese. Cool until ready to serve.

Nutrition: 261 calories; 11 g of fat; 36.3 g carbohydrates; 3.2 g of protein; 27 mg cholesterol; 242 mg of sodium

Fruit Pizza

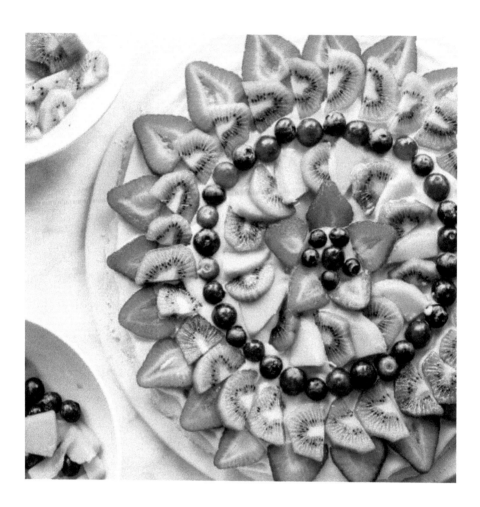

Preparation time: 30 Minutes

Servings: 8 servings

Ingredients:

- Sugar cookie dough in a cooled package of 1 oz (18 oz), cream cheese in a package of 1 (8 ounces), softened
- 1 (8 oz.) Frozen defrosted filling, defrosted, 2 cups of freshly cut strawberries
- 1/2 cup of white sugar, 1 pinch of salt
- 1 tablespoon corn flour, 2 tablespoons lemon juice, 1/2 cup orange juice
- 1/4 cup water, 1/2 teaspoon orange zest

Directions:

Preheat the oven to 175 ° C (350 ° F). Slice the cookie dough then place it on a greased pizza pan. Press the dough flat into the mold. Bake for 10 to 12 minutes. Let cool.

Soften the cream cheese in a large bowl and then stir in the whipped topping. Spread over the cooled crust. You can relax for a moment at this stage or continue to arrange the fruit.

Start with strawberries cut in half. Place them in a circle around the outer edge. Continue with the fruit of your choice by going to the center. If you use bananas, immerse them in lemon juice so that they do not get dark. Then make a sauce with a spoon on the fruit.

Combine sugar, salt, corn flour, orange juice, lemon juice, and water in a pan. Boil and stir over medium heat. Bring to the boil and cook for 1 or 2 minutes until thick. Remove from heat and add the grated orange zest. Cool, but not in place. Place on the fruit. Allow to cool for two hours, cut into quarters, and serve.

Nutrition: 535 calories; 30 g fat; 62.9 g carbohydrates; 5.5 g of protein; 49 mg cholesterol; 357 mg of sodium

Bananas Foster

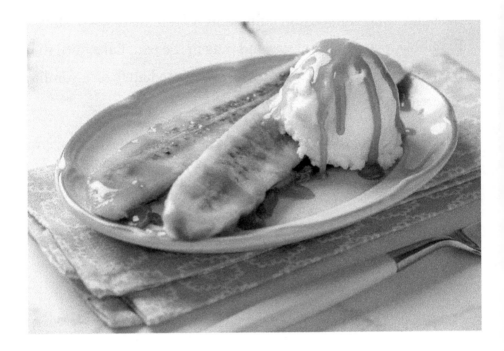

Preparation time: 5 minutes

Servings: 4 Servings

Ingredients:

- 2/3 cup dark brown sugar, 1/4 cup butter
- 3 1/2 tablespoons rum, 1 1/2 teaspoon vanilla extract
- 1/2 teaspoon of ground cinnamon
- 3 bananas, peeled and cut lengthwise and broad
- 1/4 cup coarsely chopped nuts1, vanilla ice cream

Directions:

Melt the butter in a big, deep frying pan over medium heat. Stir in sugar, rum, vanilla, and cinnamon. When the mixture starts to bubble, place the bananas and nuts in the pan. Bake until the bananas are hot, 1 to 2 minutes. Serve immediately on a vanilla ice cream.

Nutrition: 534 calories; 23.8 g of fat; 73.2 g carbohydrates; 4.6 g of protein; 60 mg cholesterol; 146 mg of sodium.

Cranberry Orange Cookies

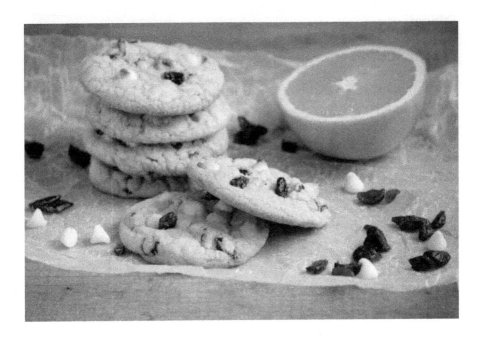

Preparation time: 20 Minutes

Servings: 48 servings

Ingredients:

- 1 cup of soft butter, 1 cup of white sugar
- 1/2 cup brown sugar, 1 egg, 1 teaspoon grated orange peel
- 2 tablespoons orange juice, 2 1/2 cups flour, 1/2 teaspoon baking powder
- 1/2 teaspoon salt, 2 cups chopped cranberries, 1/2 cup chopped walnuts (optional)

- 1/2 teaspoon grated orange peel, 3 tablespoons orange juice, 1 ½ cup confectioner's sugar

Direction:

Preheat the oven to 190 ° C.

Combine butter, white sugar, and brown sugar in a large bowl until smooth. Beat the egg until everything is well mixed. Mix 1 teaspoon of orange zest and 2 tablespoons of orange juice. Mix the flour, baking powder, and salt; stir in the orange mixture. Mix the cranberries and, if used, the nuts until well distributed. Place the dough per rounded soup spoon on ungreased baking trays. The cookies must be placed at least 2 inches away.

Bake in the preheated oven for 12 to 14 minutes, until the edges are golden brown. Remove baking trays to cool on racks.

Get a small bowl, mix 1/2 teaspoon of orange peel, 3 tablespoons of orange juice, and icing confectionery ingredients. Spread over cooled cookies. Let's act

Nutrition: 110 calories; 4.8 g fat; 16.2 g carbohydrates; 1.1 g of protein; 14 mg of cholesterol; 67 mg of sodium.

Key Pie Vill

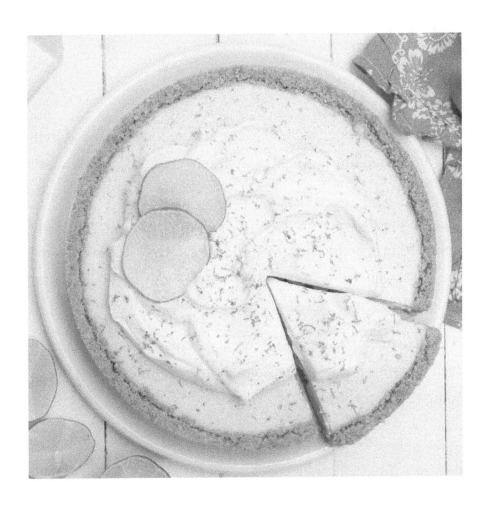

Preparation time: 15 minutes

Servings: 8 Servings

Ingredients:

- 1 (9 inches) prepared graham cracker crust
- 3 cups of sweetened condensed milk

- 1/2 cup sour cream
- 3/4 cup lime juice
- 1 tablespoon grated lime zest

Directions:

Preheat the oven to 175 ° C (350 ° F).

Combine the condensed milk, sour cream, lime juice, and lime zest in a medium bowl. Mix well and pour into the graham cracker crust.

Bake in the preheated oven for 5 to 8 minutes until small hole bubbles burst on the surface of the cake. DON'T BROWN! Cool the cake well before serving. Decorate with lime slices and whipped cream if desired.

Nutrition: 553 calories, 20.5 grams of fat; 84.7 g carbohydrates; 10.9 g of protein; 45 mg cholesterol; 324 mg of sodium

Rhubarb Strawberry Crunch

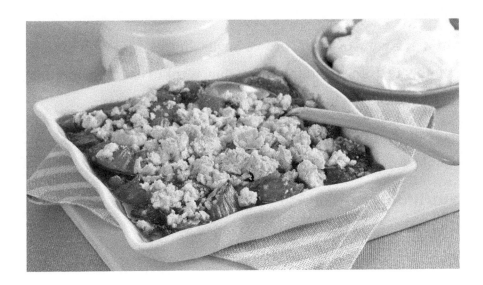

Preparation time: 15 Minutes

Servings: 18 servings

Ingredients:

- 1 cup of white sugar, 3 tablespoons all-purpose flour
- 3 cups of fresh strawberries cut into slices
- 3 cups of rhubarb cut into cubes
- 1 1/2 cup flour, 1 cup packed brown sugar
- 1 cup butter, 1 cup oatmeal

Directions:

Preheat the oven to 190 ° C.

Combine white sugar, 3 tablespoons flour, strawberries and rhubarb in a large bowl. Place the mixture in a 9 x 13-inch baking dish.

Mix 1 1/2 cups of flour, brown sugar, butter, and oats until a crumbly texture is obtained. You may want to use a blender for this. Crumble the mixture of rhubarb and strawberry.

Bake in the preheated oven for 45 minutes or until crispy and light brown.

Nutrition: 253 calories; 10.8 g fat; 38.1 g carbohydrates; 2.3 g of protein; 27 mg cholesterol; 78 mg of sodium.

Banana Dessert with Chocolate Chips

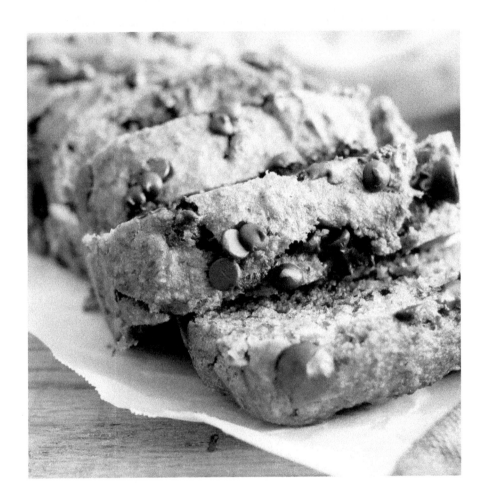

Preparation time: 20 minutes

Servings: 24 servings

Ingredients:

- 2/3 cup white sugar, 3/4 cup butter

- 2/3 cup brown sugar, 1 egg, beaten loose
- 1 teaspoon vanilla extract, 1 cup of banana puree
- 1 3/4 cup flour, 2 teaspoons baking powder
- 1/2 teaspoon of salt, 1 cup of semi-sweet chocolate chips

Directions:

Preheat the oven to 175 ° C (350 ° F). Grease and bake a 10 x 15-inch jelly baking pan.

Beat the butter, white sugar, and brown sugar in a large bowl until light. Beat the egg and vanilla. Fold in the banana puree: mix baking powder, flour, and salt in another bowl. Stir the flour mixture into the butter mixture. Stir in the chocolate chips. Spread in the prepared pan.

Bake in the preheated oven for 20 minutes until the mixture is tender. Cool before cutting into squares.

Nutrition: 174 calories; 8.2 g fat; 25.2 g carbohydrates; 1.7 g of protein; 23 mg of cholesterol; 125 mg of sodium.

Apple Pie Filling

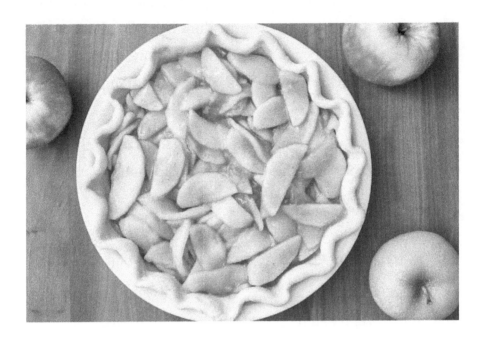

Preparation time: 20 Minutes

Servings: 40 servings

Ingredients:

- 18 cups chopped apples, 3 tablespoons lemon juice
- 10 cups of water, 4 1/2 cups of white sugar
- 1 cup corn flour
- 2 teaspoons of ground cinnamon, 1 teaspoon of salt
- 1/4 teaspoon ground nutmeg

Directions:

Mix apples with lemon juice in a large bowl and set aside. Pour the water in a Dutch oven over medium heat. Combine sugar, corn flour, cinnamon, salt, and nutmeg in a bowl. Add to water, mix well, and bring to the boil. Cook for 2 minutes with continuous stirring.

Add the apples and bring to the boil again. Lower the heat, cover, and simmer until the apples are soft about 6 to 8 minutes. Allow cooling for 30 minutes.

Pour into five freezer containers and leave a 1/2-inch free space. Cool to room temperature for no longer than one and a half hours.

Seal and freeze. It can be stored for up to 12 months.

Nutrition: 129 calories; 0.1 g fat; 33.4 g carbohydrates; 0.2 g of protein; 0 mg of cholesterol; 61 mg of sodium.

Ice cream Sandwich Dessert

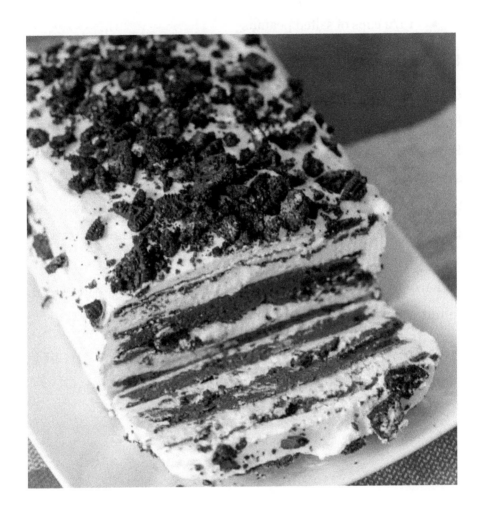

Preparation time: 20 minutes

Servings: 12 Servings

Ingredients:

- 22 ice cream sandwiches

- Frozen whipped topping in 16 oz container, thawed
- 1 Jar (12 oz) Caramel ice cream
- 1 1/2 cups of salted peanuts

Directions:

Cut a sandwich with ice in two. Place a whole sandwich and a half sandwich on a short side of a 9 x 13-inch baking dish. Repeat this until the bottom is covered, alternate the full sandwich, and the half sandwich. Spread half of the beaten topping. Pour the caramel over it. Sprinkle with half the peanuts. Repeat the layers with the rest of the ice cream sandwiches, whipped cream, and peanuts. The pan is full. Cover and freeze for up to 2 months. Remove from the freezer 20 minutes before serving. Cut into squares.

Nutrition: 559 calories 28.8 g fat; 70.9 g carbohydrates; 10 g of protein; 37 mg of cholesterol; 322 mg of sodium.

Conclusion

In the Mediterranean diet there is no calorie count, no fasting and no elimination of whole food groups. The main idea is good balance and moderation. Balance your food intake well and emphasize those that can be consumed in abundance. Don't overdo it - prepare small portions and consume in moderation.

Everyone should think about how the Mediterranean diet can best be tailored to their lifestyle and personal taste. Focus your menu on the foods this diet contains and focus on the foods you like the most. Sweet treats are not excluded, but it is desirable that they are consumed less frequently and in smaller quantities.

Be physically active by aiming for at least 30 minutes a day or 150 minutes a week. Maintain a healthy weight. Drink alcohol in moderation and give up cigarettes.